M.A.N.U.S.C.R.I.P.T.

10 Principles to a better you

by
Augusta D. Hathaway

This book is dedicated to my son Augusta DeJuan
Hathaway Jr.

Thank you for allowing me the opportunity to be your
father. You bring me much joy and a fresh wave of purpose
and motivation.
Papa Lion loves his baby lion ROAR!

INTRODUCTION

M.A.N.U.S.C.R.I.P.T. is a 10-principle daily guide to aid in the development and improvement of men. Just in case you have not noticed, the first three letters are M.A.N. Men have always had a responsible role since the beginning of time, to be leaders in their homes, jobs, teams, countries, and other positions of leadership. In the Bible, God gave Adam the responsibility of naming each animal and he also placed Adam in charge of the Garden of Eden. In fact, Eve was even made from Adam's rib. As time evolved, men took on the roles of protector, provider, hunter, and gatherer. Before the integration of military forces, it was men who fought in the famous wars and battles we have all read about. Just to clarify, this book is not intended to bash women or imply that women are the weaker sex, for women have important roles in every facet of life. This is not a book to prove Biblical or religious principles, or to pit men against women. My intent is to bring back to light the significance and importance of a MAN, while providing both biblical and practical tools to implement. Providing you daily encouragement to become a better man, not only for yourself, but also for those who are a part of your life. Has the quality of men weakened? Have men forgotten the value and pride of being a man? These are some questions I have pondered while noticing the value of men significantly decreasing over the years. Men have become less responsible, less protective, more selfish, and even unfit. Men, we cannot allow the norms of today's society for men to become the normalization of manhood. We were born to be strong, courageous leaders, providers, and protectors. You are a Man, and you were born with a purpose to change the world. Through many reads, podcasts, conferences, and other forms of education, I have developed 10 principles that men have practiced for centuries, bringing much success and purpose to men over the years. These 10 principles are to be implemented and practiced each day of your life. Initially, you may not implement all these principles, but remember, it's all about progress. Like the saying goes, Rome was not built in a day.

To help you along your journey of becoming a better man, journal the results each day you practice each of these principles. It's okay if you start off practicing 1, 3, or even 6 of these principles. As stated before, the goal is progression. Progression to the point where it becomes second nature. Personally, I too did not initially implement each of these principles, but over time and with persistence, these 10 principles have become a daily routine. I am excited that you have selected this book to better yourself, and I have no doubt that you will climb too even greater heights in your career, family, and personal endeavors. Let's begin your journey to greatness as we dive into the MANUSCRIPT.

Principle 1: <u>Meditation</u>

Everything whether good or bad, starts with a thought. If we meditate on something long enough it can become a reality in our life. So, it is important that our thoughts are steering the direction in which we want our life to go. As men, we often forget to take daily time to meditate. Whether if it's through prayer, affirmations, or even just quite time, it is vital that we take some portion of our day and simply get some quite time to ourselves. Many of us wake up, go to work, and come home to our family which then demands our attention. In between those responsibilities we squeeze in gym time, mowing the lawn, kids practices and other task that require our attention. Yet often do we squeeze in time for meditation? Oxford languages defines meditation as a written or spoken discourse expressing considered thoughts on a subject. More than often, men tend to take their work and work problems home which results in limited emotional capacity that we can provide to our families. Other areas include our relationships or extracurricular activities we may be involved in. Many studies have shown that meditation can decrease stress, increase creativity, improve self-confidence and overall managing negative emotions. You may be asking "what should I mediate about and how often should I meditate?". Here are some suggestions to help you with this principle of meditation.

1). Meditate every day for a minimum of 5-10 minutes at a time. I suggest this time range because I feel it's a great time range to start and build upon, especially if you have not performed a lot of meditation. As your able to meditate undistracted, add more time to your meditation session. Regarding frequency, begin with one session daily and add more sessions as you feel led to.

2). Meditate in the early part of the morning, late evenings, lunch breaks or driving to and from work. I suggest these times because these are usually times when we are often alone. If none of these suggestions work for you, then find some time and space where you can spend 5-10 minutes a day to meditate.

3). Meditate outdoors as much as possible. There is something about the freshness of air, soft grass, sand under our feet or hearing the soothing sounds of crashing waves. Many refer to this connection as biophilia. We are nature so spend time with nature.

4). Keep a small journal for reflections of thoughts. Many of my greatest ideas came because of meditation sessions. In fact, this book is a result of a meditation session. Hundreds of thoughts and ideas come across our mind daily and many times we simply disregard them. The part is that if we act upon just one of the ideas, it could be the ticket to changing your life financially and generationally. That's why it is important to log the thoughts and ideas we encounter daily. Todays it so easy because everyone has a cell phone which has a notes app in which you can write down your thoughts. Write them down as quickly as possible and don't wait because as you prolong, you run the risk of forgetting the idea or thought you had.

Here are 8 questions that you can use to assist with your meditation. Feel free to add to this initial 8 questions as you implement meditation into your daily life.

1). What is your life purpose?

2). Are you taking steps to fulfilling your purpose?

3). In what area can you self-improve?

4). How was your day at work? Good or Bad

5). Are you taking your work problems home?

6). How are you managing negative emotions?

7). How are you impacting your wife, family, significant other, or children?

8). What do YOU want out of life?

As we conclude with principle 1, begin to think of ways to implement meditation into your daily routine. Remember everything starts with a thought and we are biproducts of our thoughts and actions. So, make sure the thoughts we meditate upon are the thought we want manifested in our lives to becoming a better MAN.

"It is indeed a radical act of love just to sit down and be quiet for a time by yourself"

– Jon Kabat-Zinn-

Principle 2: <u>A</u>ct of Kindness

Today, we are filled with a world full of selfish, self-centered, ambitious people. I remember growing up; my parents would teach me several principles about being kind to people, but particularly two principles stood out. One was the golden rule: "Treat people the way you want to be treated." Secondly, "Help someone whenever you have the ability to help them." Those two principles, which my parents instilled in me, have carried, and assisted me over the course of my life. There was a time when I used to be judgmental towards less fortunate people. It wasn't until I became homeless that I understood that any given day, at any given time, for any given reason, a person's life can drastically change for better or for worse. It wasn't until I was wrongfully terminated from my job that I understood the families that need government assistance to keep food on the table and a roof over their heads. Experience will quickly humble the proud. It will also make you sympathize with people who may be down on their luck. As for me, it led me to perform more acts of kindness towards people. Many times, we focus just on ourselves. We say things like, "I want a raise," "I deserve better," or "What about me?" Yet we forget that even though we may be going through a challenge, there is always someone going through a tougher challenge. Many times, it is so hard to unravel who may be going through a challenge because people do such a great job of disguising their pains. In a society of social media likes and follows, we often give off this false impression that our life is so perfect, and everything is just dandy. Yet the reality is that this world is filled with hurting people. People that are afraid or do not want to reach out for help. The solution is that we possess the key to change someone's life just by doing a small act of kindness. One act of kindness could save a person from committing suicide. One act of kindness can boost a person's confidence to start a business. One act of kindness can motivate an individual to go back to school to get their diploma. We never know the effects that our act of kindness can have on someone. Whenever we plant a seed good or bad in someone's life, we always reap a bigger harvest than what we planted. For example, if I plant a single apple seed, that single apple seed over time will produce hundreds of apples. To the same effect, the seeds we plant in other people's life will soon blossom and show in our own life; so be sure the seeds you are planting are the seeds you want to be exhibited in your life. What are some ways in which you can exhibit Acts of Kindness? Below are a few questions to help you along with this principle.

1). How can you show an act of kindness at home or at work?

2). Who comes to your mind when you think of performing an Act of Kindness? Why?

3). How can you exhibit Acts of Kindness within your community?

4). Have you ever had the opportunity to perform an Act of Kindness and chose not to? Why?

"Don't judge each day by the harvest you reap but by the seed you plant."

-Robert Louis Stevenson-

"Treat everyone with respect"
-Hal Luther- NFL Strength Coach

Principle 3: <u>N</u>ix Negativity

Nothing disrupts a good day more than having it tainted by hours of pointless and depressing drama from someone else. While I'm always willing to lend an ear, if every interaction with someone brings negative vibes, I reserve the right to end the conversation abruptly. While it's common to feel obligated to listen and solve others' problems, it's essential to recognize that we're not responsible for everyone else's issues, just as they're not responsible for ours. Each of us is responsible for navigating life's challenges while prioritizing internal and external tranquility. Negative emotions not only harm us emotionally but also impact our health, weakening the immune system, leading to chronic illnesses, and reducing lifespan. Therefore, it's crucial to prioritize maintaining happiness at all costs, as our health and life depend on it. This underscores the importance of what and who we choose to focus our attention on.

What to focus on:

While it's important to stay informed about local and global issues, much of the information circulated is negative. Consuming negative news multiple times, a day can overwhelm us. Similarly, interacting with consistently negative individuals can drain us emotionally and physically. Regardless of life's challenges, it's essential to consciously surround ourselves with positivity and joy.

Here are some tips for maintaining a positive environment and well-being:

1. Be comfortable spending time alone temporarily.
2. Accept that not everyone will support you.

3. Look for the silver lining in every negative situation.

4. Negativity is contagious and draining so protect your personal space.

"You just can't live in that negative way. Make way for the positive day."

-Bob Marley-

Principle 4: <u>U</u>se your words to Uplift

I am pretty sure we have all heard the phrase "Sticks and Stones may break my bones, but words can never hurt me." That by far is one of the most fabricated statements ever made. Words can shape the direction in which our life can go, either positively or negatively. It still amazes me how people utilize their words to the extent that they don't even realize why negative events have come to pass in their life. How often have we heard or even said these quotes: "This is impossible", "I'm too small", "I'm too big", "I don't have enough education", "I did not grow up in the best environments". Although all these statements may be true, verbally if we change our words, we have the power to change our circumstances. Let's look at these few examples of how people used their words and their outcomes:

"And God said, let there be light: and there was light." (Genesis 1:3),

"There's something within me that moves me to become the heavyweight champion of the world,". "And I won't stop until I satisfy this thirst within me." (George Foreman) 2x Boxing Heavyweight Champion of the World

"I'll probably be popped off by some looney." On December 8,1980, John Lennon tragically died when he was shot five times.

This list can go on and on, but I think you get the picture. As men, it's important to be self-conscious of how we utilize our words not only towards others but also ourselves. I cannot stress enough that the biggest fan of yourself needs to be you. There is something very effective intrinsically when you speak positive words over yourself. Those words begin to take seed within your spirit and when you persistently say those positive words over yourself, you will start to live out what you are saying. This is not only a spiritual law but also a natural law. Spiritual because in the beginning, everything in the Earth was created from a word. The entire first chapter of Genesis God literally spoke everything into existence. Natural because we can literally speak our way into the life we want if we act upon the words we speak. Speak, Act, Produce.

This is also true when we speak into other people's life. Good or bad, the words we speak into other people can have a lasting effect. More often it's always the negative words we tend to remember the most. Take a moment and think about the time when someone said negative words about you. You can remember how old you were, where you were, even the clothes you wore. It's sad but true. As men, many of us have families and as fathers, our children will believe what we say about them. The same goes for our wife or significant other. As men, we are supposed to be the head of our house. With each day, we can set the tone for our entire household or work environment simply by speaking positive encouraging words over those around us. You never know how one simple word of encouragement can change a person's day or life. You can be that person that gives someone the motivation and encouragement they need to get over the hump. Moving forward, I want you to become more conscious of the words you are saying towards yourself and others. Start paying close attention to what people are saying around and find that individual or individuals who need words of encouragement. How will I know who needs uplifting words? I would suggest listening not only with your ear but also your intuition. A lot of times our gut instincts alert us to something good and of something bad. Just be in tune with your inner spirit, and it will guide you to people who are needing some uplifting words. Our society is filled with hurting people and as men, we can be a light in a dark, hurting world. Let's begin to uplift the spirit of people by speaking positive words to everyone we come across. It may feel weird at first, but over time you will become more confident in this task. Remember, you don't have to encourage them with an entire sermon, just something simple such as "Be great today", "You are awesome", "Have a productive day", "You will change the world". Simple words but effective.

Below are a few tasks in which I want you to begin practicing weekly:

1. Become more self-conscious of the words you speak.

2. Say 5 positive words over yourself, family, co-workers, and other important people in your life as often as you can.

3. Find one person a day and speak positive words over them. This can be done verbally or electronically.

4. The last five minutes before you go to bed each night, say 1-2 uplifting words about yourself and if possible, those living with you (Wife, kids, girlfriend, etc.).

"Life and death are in the power of the tongue and those who love it shall eat its fruit"

Proverbs-18:21

Principle 5: <u>S</u>elf-Defense Training

Although each of these principles is important, this principle, in my opinion, is one of the most important of the ten. As men, we have a great responsibility to be protectors—protectors of ourselves, our families, and our country. It boggles my mind to see so many men's inability to defend themselves, let alone someone else. Now, I am not saying that you should train to be the next Rambo or Bruce Lee. I am simply saying that self-defense training should be a skill that men should practice on a weekly, if not daily, basis. There are many tools through which men can acquire a level of self-defense training to the point of at least being able to defend themselves in a street fight. For example, one of the most popular forms of self-defense training is Ju-Jitsu. Ju-Jitsu is a great martial art to engage in. It is primarily ground fighting, but its techniques can be utilized while standing, sitting, and in other anatomical positions. Many Ju-Jitsu dojos offer various levels of classes based on experience (Beginner, Intermediate, Advanced). The pace at which the classes are taught makes it easy for any participant to retain the information. The best thing about Ju-Jitsu is that it has been proven to be a highly effective martial art and has saved the lives of many people since its existence. I recommend pairing Ju-Jitsu with some form of striking course such as Muay Thai, Boxing, Kickboxing, or Karate. By doing so, you will become more well-rounded in your self-defense training. Having the ability to defend yourself on your feet and on the ground makes you a more lethal man.

The second form of self-defense training I recommend is learning some form of weapons training. Weapons include knives, guns, sticks, and other apparatuses for which you can become legally trained and certified for self-defense purposes. It is important that you receive proper instruction on the utilization of these weapons because they can be very dangerous and deadly. We have all seen instances in the news in which individuals utilize weapons for self-defense, only to later discover that the utilization of their weapons was not legally justified. The keyword here is "legally." I stress the word "legally" because not having the proper knowledge of when and when not to use your weapon can lead to serious ramifications such as jail time or possibly fatally harming someone. I am not here to promote one weapon over another. I am simply saying to get the proper training in a weapon that you feel comfortable using for self-defense purposes.

Here are some tips to assist you in your self-defense training:

1. Find a local Ju-Jitsu school or Mixed Martial Arts (MMA) school. If you can find a school that offers multiple martial arts training, that's a plus.
2. Stay consistent with your martial arts training. Gradually increase your frequency as you become more confident in your skill set. Remember, even a black belt begins as a white belt.
3. Find a weapons course led by a certified instructor.
4. Participate in as many refresher courses as possible. Remember, habits are not habits unless you constantly practice them.
5. Know the weapons laws in your state and surrounding areas. Remember, laws and rules change constantly, so it's crucial to stay up to date.
6) When training in martial arts or with weapons, always prioritize safety not only for yourself, but also for your training partners.

You will discover that as you consistently engage in more martial arts, your physique and confidence will improve. As men, we are called to be protectors, so take the necessary steps to position yourself to be a protector in the likelihood of facing conflict. Be ready and always stay ready!

"Take things as they are. Punch when you have to punch. Kick when you have to kick." - Bruce Lee -

Principle 6: Cash Flow

Ironically, this principle comes directly after speaking about men being protectors. Cash flow follows it. I am baffled by how many men do not take the time weekly to manage their finances. Some of you may argue that money is not an important element of manhood, yet I beg to differ. As men, it is important to provide for our families and to provide for our families, it takes money. Even as a single man, it takes money to pay for your living expenses and other necessities for everyday living. Two basic financial principles every man should follow to maintain or improve their cash flow:

1) ***Create a monthly budget that allows you to see exactly where your money is going each pay period***: Too often, we do not have the slightest clue as to where our money is going. Bills, monthly subscriptions, outings, and other daily endeavors eat away at our bank accounts, yet many men only manage their money by checking their daily ledger to ensure no overdraft has occurred. You're probably laughing because at some point, we have all been guilty of this. The reality is that having no budget is irresponsible. I get it; it can take a lot of time in addition to another task in your already busy schedule. Ask yourself, are you stewarding your money to the best of your ability? If you answered yes, then congratulations. Continue to improve your stewardship of your finances. If you answered no, then you may want to consider building a monthly budget sheet to assist with your cash flow. Being able to visually see where your money is disbursed can help you make the necessary changes to better steward your money. At the end of this book, I have provided a budget spreadsheet, which has assisted me over the years to better budget my

finances. It has drastically made a tremendous impact on the decisions of how and where I spend my money.

2) *Save:* How many times have you heard the phrase, "pay yourself first"? I have heard it pretty much my entire adult life. Although hearing the phrase became redundant, this statement holds so much truth. You are the one who puts in the work; you are the one that must sacrifice day in and day out, so pay yourself first. Not the government, not the loans, no one or nothing but yourself first. Even if it is only a hundred bucks a pay period. That money which you are putting away will one day come in handy. Why, may you ask? Because accidents are going to happen; it's inevitable. Home repairs, car repairs, medical expenses, the list goes on and on. Yet, it's these unexpected expenses that often-put people into a financial crisis. The best way to tackle these crises is to have some money set aside when one does occur. Although I am no financial advisor, I recommend at least paying yourself at least 10-15% of your paycheck. If this number is too high for you, then do what you can. Something is better than nothing. Doing nothing is not being a smart manager of your finances, nor is it being a leader of your home. As men, it is important that we lead, especially in finances.

3) *Investing:* is the next important factor of cash flow. If you continue living, you will get old, which means your body gradually slows down and working a nine-to-five won't be as feasible. Therefore, we need to invest in things that generate cash flow without necessarily requiring physical work. I am not going to make recommendations about what you should invest in, but there is a lot of information available for you to research which provides ideas for avenues to generate passive income. The bottom line is that no one is going to care for yourself or your family as much as you do. So, as men, it is important that we position ourselves financially, which

will, in the long haul, position us better in life. Strategically positioning yourself financially all starts with:

1. Getting on a budget

2. Saving Money

3. Investing in areas that will generate cash flow (passive income).

Below are some recommendations to increase your financial literacy:

1. Get a financial advisor.

2. Listen to financial podcasts for 30 minutes a day.

3. Attend financial workshops when possible.

4. GET ON A BUDGET.

"Good Money management is Good Life management."

\- Author Unknown –

Principle 7: <u>Read</u>

Knowledge is key, and Ignorance is what we don't know. As men, many of us have a prideful spirit. We tend to think we know everything and that our way is the best and only way. Our ways are sometimes dumb and not efficient, leading to wasted time and money. If we are not careful, it could lead to more serious losses such as a job, wife, or family. That's why it is important to always continue to educate yourself. One of the best ways is through reading. Reading is a great way to stimulate your mind, because so much hidden knowledge lies between the lines of a book. Before there was technology, there were only books. Today, reading is almost a lost art due to the advancement of technology. The good thing is that we can still utilize technology as a tool for reading. If you're like me, I prefer to read along while the author reads (via technology) as I follow along. Yet sometimes I like to read the traditional way, with a bookmark, pen, and highlighter.

Although the traditional reading form tends to be outdated, I have written some of the best notes, which were revealed to me through my intuition. I highly encourage you to read the traditional way as much as possible. You will discover creativity, revelation, and wisdom begin to flow from you like rivers of water. I encourage you that as those thoughts come to you, write them down in a journal and put the date on which the thought came to your mind. Although the same has occurred whenever I read via technology, the mental and spiritual connection was just not the same as traditional reading. Reading allows us to return to that childlike spirit by opening our imagination and beginning to dream again. It has been said that when a man stops dreaming, then he begins to mentally die. The Bible reads in Hosea 4:6 "My people perish for lack of knowledge". One way to gain knowledge is through reading. As men, we love to grow our muscles and our bank accounts, but we must also grow our minds. Personal development is a key factor in the continuous growth of manhood. By choosing this book, you are taking steps towards your personal development as a man. I encourage you to not only read this book but also other books to assist you along your journey to becoming a better version of yourself. Below are some suggestions and recommended for you:

1. Read one to two books per month.
2. Read as many books as possible from these categories: finances, health, mental thinking, leadership, relationships, and self-defense.
3. When possible, choose pages over electronic reads.
4. Read in 20–30-minute blocks to reduce concentration loss.
5. Encourage other men to read with you (e.g., Men's group).
6. Read in places where you can focus and hear with your inner ear (e.g., Park, library).
7. Write down what you hear within your spirit.

"A reader lives a thousand lives before he dies... The man who never reads lives only one."
- George R.R. Martin-

Principle 8: Influence others

Our society is filled with so many followers and only a handful of leaders. Every day I watch men neglect the trueness of themselves to fit in with the crowd. This is not only weak but also reveals one's inability to influence others. Before I go further with this principle, whenever I use the word influence, I mean positively influencing others in a way which challenges them too daily better themselves. When I hear the word influence, I think of great men such as Martin Luther King Jr., Billy Graham, Bob Marley, and Jesus Christ. These men left such an impact on the world that they are still greatly referenced to this very day. What made these men so special? Why were they followed by so many people? My guess is that these men were: 1) They stayed true to themselves. Simply put, these men did not change their beliefs or values to please people. They stood firm in their values and principles regardless of criticism they may have encountered. Men of influence tend to have a special connection with people to the point that people believe every word which comes from the influencer's mouth. More importantly, they aid in the personal development of people. 2) Men of Influence are not afraid to be alone. Many great influencers tend to be loners, meaning that they have no problem being by themselves. Nor do they need the approval of other people. This is a huge factor, especially if you want to be a man of influence. As men, being alone can be a positive situation. The reason being is that alone time can minimize distractions, which ultimately heightens your focus and ability to think and hear much clearer. Each of us has a purpose in life, and it is important that we discover and fulfill our purpose. Although we all have individual purposes, your purpose is designed to help others reach their life purpose. Therefore, it is vital to daily use your gifts to positively influence others and not allow others to deter you from your life purpose.

Men of influence always follow their intuition. Whenever you have time, I recommend you briefly read about each of the influential men I mentioned earlier. Several times throughout their life, each man-made historical decisions by listening to their intuition. Yes, these men sought wise counsel from others, but sometimes your intuition strongly overpowers any advice you may receive. Often, regardless of whether the situation is good or bad, our intuition provides us the answer before we are revealed the answer. Never neglect your intuition because it can be a life changer and a life saver.

I challenge you each day in your home, workplace, or any vicinity in which you are interacting with people to focus on two things:

1. Pay attention to the people around you and identify who is the primary influencer. Is the influencer positively or negatively influencing others?
2. Who are you influencing or are you being influenced?

Being someone of great influence is no easy task, and to become a great influencer, one must be willing to take a lot of criticism and spend a lot of days as a loner. As you begin your journey to becoming a better influencer, keep those thoughts in the forefront of your mind. Know that if you stay true to yourself, accept times of loneliness, and listen to your intuition, that you are on the path to becoming someone of great influence. People, friendships, and relationships change, but your purpose also can change people. Choose your purpose over people because fulfilling your purpose will have a lasting effect on the people.

"You must be the change you wish to see in the world"
-Mahatma Gandhi-

Principle 9: Physical Fitness

If I were asked to rank these principles from one to ten, this principle would be number one on my list. Simply put, our body and our health are our most valuable assets. The better we take care of our bodies, the more productive we can be executing these 10 principles. As men, we need to set the example for ourselves, our family, and those around us, that our health and physical appearance are important standards to us. Many men have the perception that being physically fit is having bulging biceps and a sculpted six-pack. This is so far from the truth. As a lifelong fitness specialist, I can tell you firsthand that I have had hundreds of clients with bulging biceps and six-packs but were overall not physically fit. How can this be, you may wonder? Well, being physically fit requires a lot more than just lifting weights; it also revolves around cardiovascular health, diet, sleep, stress levels, and other factors that play a role in our overall fitness level. During this principle, I will discuss four areas of physical fitness that I want you to focus on to improve your overall health. I will also provide a 30-day physical fitness training chart **(see 30-Day Calendar)** for you to follow to provide you some training guidance. As usual, I will conclude with some advice and tips to assist you on your journey to becoming a more physically fit man. As mentioned earlier, here are four areas to improve your physical fitness:

1). Stop making so many excuses:
  - "I don't have time."
  - "Gym memberships are too expensive."
  - "Dad bods are in."
  - "I am not trying to become bulky."

Nothing irritates me more than hearing a man make excuses as to why he cannot maintain his fitness levels. Although physical fitness requires personal effort, it is also necessary so we can be physically useful to others. Think about it, how useful is an individual on the job if he is unable to perform the required physical tasks? This is what I mean by being men who are physically fit. Fitness is much bigger than muscle sculpting; it enables us to remain physically productive on the job, which ultimately keeps food on the table. As men, it is vital that you make time daily to incorporate physical fitness, even if it's just 20 minutes a day. Do something daily to improve your overall physical fitness. The biggest mental roadblock men have when it comes to physical fitness is that they feel all their fitness must be performed in one session. The reality is that your fitness can be spread throughout the day or week. Not to mention, fitness is not just limited to a gym. Just get creative and think outside the box. Here is an example: Tom works 10-hour shifts 3 days a week. On these days, he cannot make his one-hour gym session, so he does bodyweight exercises while at work. His routine includes 40 push-ups, 40 squats, and 40 seated or standing crunches every hour. During lunch, he walks for 10 minutes prior to eating his lunch. At the end of his work session, Tom has completed 400 push-ups, squats, seated crunches, and a 10-minute walk. This is an example of a man not making excuses but finding a way to take care of his physical health. We find time for things that are important to us, so make physical fitness an important part of your daily routine.

2). ***Don't limit physical fitness to just the gym***. Get out of your head that to maintain fitness levels, you must be in a gym. No, no, no. There are so many avenues in which you can maintain fitness levels other than the gym. The important thing is that you select something that will keep you focused, motivated, consistent, and engaged. For example, I love to participate in martial arts. It stimulates me mentally and physically. It also allows me to engage in physical activity without the redundancy of always being in a gym. I get it, gyms can be boring and monotonous, so find things that will keep you motivated but more importantly consistent in daily physical activity.

3). **Pack rather than pay**. We all have heard the saying, "You are what you eat." This statement holds a lot of truth when it comes to our physical fitness. The foods we intake not only affect us externally but also internally. As men, a lot of times we are on the go and pressed for time, which at times forces us to eat out. Now, I am not saying eating out is bad, but we want to limit the frequency of how many times we are eating out. A lot of times our food options are not the best whenever we must eat out, which is why I recommend packing your lunch daily when possible. This will allow you to better monitor your diet but also save you time and money. One of the easiest methods is to prep your breakfast and lunch for two-day splits. Here is an example: Every Sunday, Juan prepares his breakfast and lunch for the next two days (Monday, Tuesday); on Wednesday, he eats out, but that evening he prepares his breakfast and lunch for the final two workdays (Thursday, Friday). This is a method I found highly effective and easy to remain consistent. It also eliminates the amount of wasted food, which is also a waste of money. Whether you are trying to gain or lose weight, you can better monitor your food intake when packing rather than paying.

4). ***Take you're a** to sleep.*** Men, I get it! We are grinders, and we try to maximize our time because time is money! Yet, what good is that money if you croak due to a lack of sleep? As much as we hate to, we must give our body and mind a rest. It is during that rest in which our bodies and minds recover and rejuvenate. Lack of sleep is not only dangerous, but it can negatively affect our performance and open the door to many health issues. To help you monitor your sleep, I encourage you to purchase an apparatus that tracks and monitors your sleep. Many of these devices can provide in-depth information, such as the number of hours you slept, your current recovery level, and a score of your overall physical performance status for the current workday. We often sacrifice our sleep for late-night activities like sex, finishing a project, or watching a television series marathon. None of these activities are inherently bad, but they can become issues when they become consistent habits. Listen to your body when it gives you signs of fatigue. It's okay to take a rest. The work, projects, family, and friends will still be there once you awaken. You will probably be more productive after a few minutes or hours of extra sleep.

I hope you find these four areas related to fitness improvement useful and will incorporate them into your daily routine. Below are seven other points I advise each of my clients during their personal physical fitness journey. Utilize the 30-day fitness calendar as much as possible and build your own calendar once you feel comfortable doing so. If you have any medical issues, I recommend checking with your physician before engaging in any physical activity. Lastly, treat your body as a temple because you only get one.

1. Don't compare your fitness journey to others. Remember, it's you versus you!

2. Try to increase your sleep by 30 extra minutes a night or take a nap (20-30 minutes) during the day. Either way, prioritize rest!

3. Increase your water intake. Water not only hydrates our bodies but also aids in flushing toxins from our bodies.

4. Engage in a variety of physical activities to reduce boredom and inconsistency.

5. The scale does not always show physical improvements.

6. Maintain consistency.

7. Remember, whatever you put in your mouth will eventually show externally."

You can find more great workouts and tips in my other publication titled "Special Forces Fitness Training" Gym Free workouts which provides over 300 exercises and workouts you can perform in the comfort of your own home.

"I hate working out, but damn I look good in this mirror"
-Augusta D. Hathaway"

Principle:10 Thankfulness

I complained that my home was too small until I saw a homeless man. I complained that my car was too old until I saw a family walking in the rain. I used to think I was too short until I saw a man without legs, and I used to think the world was an ugly place until I met a man who could not see. We all have areas in our life that we wish were better, yet even in our current situations, there is always something to be thankful for. To be thankful is to be happy and content with our current circumstances. The universe always seems to provide a level of abundance to those who are always expressing an attitude of thankfulness. Take a moment and think of someone you know who is always expressing an attitude of thankfulness. They always seem to be happy, flourishing in life, having healthy relationships, and pleasant to be around. It goes back to point number 3: no one likes to be around a negative person. Vibes are contagious, so accept only positive vibes.

Whenever I hear the word "Thankful," I think of this word as two-fold. "Thank" is to be in a state of appreciation. "Ful" is to be filled. When combined, it means to be filled with appreciation. During my life, I have been on both ends of the spectrum, experiencing massive success and lows in life. It was not until I encountered the lows that I became full of appreciation for the seasons of success. Life is like a seesaw; it's a constant up and down ride. The great thing is when you maintain an attitude of thankfulness even during the low seasons, sooner or later you will rise into your season of success. Below is a task I want you to perform whenever you're alone and can reflect on five areas: *Family, Home, Relationships, Health, and Job*. For each of these categories, I want you to write down and confess five things you are thankful for in each category. The sole purpose is that whenever you are at a low point in this seesaw ride, we call life, you can reflect on the thankful notes you wrote for each category. Each day you're alive, be grateful for life, for that means God still has a purpose and plan for you to fulfill on Earth. Don't go through life dwelling on past failures; instead, take that negative experience and find something to be thankful for.

As we come to the end of this book, I am thankful for each of you for taking the time to read my book, but more importantly, investing in bettering yourself. All I ask in return, is to share this knowledge with others to encourage personal growth in others around the world. Revisit this book as much as possible and practice these principles often. As stated earlier, start with one or two principles each day and continue to add more daily until it becomes second nature. Remember, you are a MAN, and God has placed a lot of responsibility and assignments on men while on Earth. The good news is that He has also provided the necessary tools to accomplish these assignments. You will encounter times of discouragement but press on. Your life depends on it, your family depends on it, and your country depends on it! Let's continue to keep the pride and prestige of being a MAN and train up the next generation of men. Be the man God called and expects you to be.

"Faithfulness in seasons of sorrow is followed by fruitfulness in seasons of harvest."

- Bishop Dale C. Bronner-

PERSONAL BUGDET FORM

BUDGET & DEBT REDUCTION	Check 1	Check 2	Other Pay
Tithes			
Q1. SELF PAY			
Savings			
Emergency Fund			
Retirement, IRA,etc			
Q2.-NECCESITIES			
Rent/Mortgage( )			
HOA ( )			
Grocery ( )			
Gas( )			
Cell phone ( )			
Car Insurance ( )			
Electric( )			
Water( )			
Q3- DEBTS			
Balance Remainder			

Example: You can plug and play as you choose

30 DAY PHYSICAL TRAINING CALENDAR

SUNDAY	MONDAY	TUESDAY	WEDNESDAY	THURSDAY	FRIDAY	SATURDAY
30 minute Outdoor walk	Weight Training Total body	30 minute Bike Ride	Rest & Recovery	20 minute Meditation	Martial Arts Training	YOGA
Rest & Recovery	Martial Arts Training	Weight Training Total body	YOGA	Weight Training Total body	20 minute Meditation	30-minute cardio (Your choice)
30-minute Bike Ride	YOGA	Weight Training Total body	20 minute Meditation	Martial Arts Training	Weight Training Total body	Rest & Recovery
Rest & Recovery	Weight Training Total body	Martial Arts Training	30-minute Outdoor walk	YOGA	Weight Training Total body	Martial Arts Training
					Weight Training Total body	YOGA

Example: This is an illustration of a 30-day training routine. Plug in your favorite physical activities for each day of the month.

About the Author

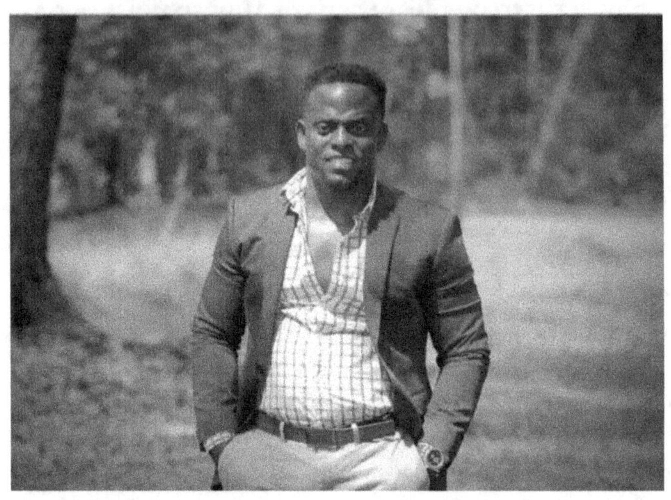

Augusta DeJuan Hathaway is a man that has been gifted with so many talents. He is a father, fighter, fitness expert, author but more importantly a follower of Jesus Christ. His passion has always been to assist people improve their overall health and lifestyle. Spending the last 15 years assisting men and women of the United States military in physical fitness. His commitment to enhancing soldier fitness has identified him as one of the top professionals in his career field and receiving many notable awards for his service.

He was born and raised in Murfreesboro, Tennessee, where he excelled in both football and track. He later continued his football career at Maryville College in which he also earned his Bachelor of Arts Degree in Physical Education. Pursing further education, he graduated from the University of Hawaii-Manoa with a Master's Degree in Kinesiology. During his college years, Augusta DeJuan discovered his gift for writing. Since then, he has published several works. His first publication Special Forces Fitness Training: *Gym Free Workouts*, has been translated in multiple languages and sold hundreds of copies globally. In his leisure time, he enjoys martial arts, dancing, cooking and outdoor activities. He believes the secret to a long fulfilling life is to be healthy and happiness. Augusta DeJuan's goal is to continue sharing his life journey and to inspire others around the world find their purpose and passion.